MASSAGE FOR HORSES

by

Mary Bromiley FCSP, RPT(USA), SRP

Illustrations by
Carole Vincer

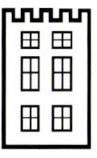

KENILWORTH PRESS

First published in the UK in 1996 by
Kenilworth Press, an imprint of Quiller Publishing Ltd

© The Kenilworth Press Limited 1996
Reprinted 1997, 2000, 2006

All rights reserved. No part of this publication
may be reproduced, stored in a retrieval system, or
transmitted in any form or by any means, electronic,
mechanical, photocopying, recording or otherwise,
without the written permission of the publisher.

British Library Cataloguing in Publication Data
A catalogue record for this book is available from the British Library.

ISBN   1-872082-87-4
       978-1-872082-87-5

Printed in Great Britain by Halstan & Co. Ltd

KENILWORTH PRESS
An imprint of Quiller Publishing Ltd
Wykey House, Wykey, Shrewsbury, SY4 1JA
tel: 01939 261616 fax: 01939 261606
website: www.kenilworthpress.co.uk

Important note
In the Great Britian it is a legal offence for any person to practise massage on an animal owned by another person without the permission of a veterinary surgeon, normally the veterinary surgeon who would attend the animal in question. (Veterinary Surgeons Act, 1966)
   It is assumed that persons practising the described massage techniques are fully aware of the risks associated with work around horses.
   The author and publisher are not responsible for any injury sustained by persons attempting to massage, neither can they be held responsible for any injury resulting from the inappropriate use of massage.

CONTENTS

MASSAGE FOR HORSES

4 Introduction
5 Surface anatomy
6 Lymphatic and circulatory systems
8 Massage techniques
11 Massage equipment
12 Body massage
16 The pleasure horse
17 Dressage
18 Endurance riding
19 Driving
20 Show jumping
21 Cross-country
22 Ice massage
23 Teaching and strengthening the hands
24 Indications for massage

Introduction

Massage is a method of influencing the soft tissue masses of a body, utilising varied hand techniques, each technique requiring the hands of the masseur to perform in a prescribed manner.

These techniques bear French names, for the French were the first to transcribe translations of 3000-year-old Chinese manuscripts.

Today massage is often categorised as an alternative therapy, a method to be employed following injury. It is possible to enhance the recovery of damaged tissue utilising massage *but* the real place of massage is: **applied pre-activity** to prepare the body for exercise, thereby enhancing performance and preventing injury; and **employed following activity** to reduce muscle fatigue and ensure a rapid return to normal.

Effects of massage
• **Mechanical:** It enhances the passage of the waste-laden venous blood as it passes through the venous complex toward the body centre.

It also influences the movement of the alternative waste collector and body defence fluid, lymph.

The clearance of waste from muscles promotes general health.

• **Reflex:** It promotes relaxation. The hands, passing over the skin surface, trigger impulses in small superficially sited nerve receptors. These signals, when received in the brain, cause a local muscle relaxation.

This effect is *not* achieved unless the massage is applied in a monotonous repetitive manner with no sudden variations of speed or pressure.

• **Stimulatory:** The application of the hands in a brisk, rapid manner achieves stimulation, particularly using hacking or clapping techniques.

• **Massage does not develop muscle strength. It is *not* a substitute for exercise.**

Surface Anatomy

The Surface

The **skin** is the largest organ of the body, providing a protective outer covering for the entire body mass. It has a major role in temperature regulation, and is richly endowed with neural receptors (nerve endings) of many types. Some receptors can be influenced by massage, promoting relaxation and dilating and/or constricting superficial blood vessels.

Massage is applied by exerting pressure over the exterior surface of the body, using sufficient compression to affect the structures lying beneath. These include:

- **Muscles** – the main organs of locomotion.
- **Tendons** – extensions of muscles, sited mostly in the distal limbs.
- **Ligaments** – specialist bands of tissue primarily utilised to hold the bones in their appropriate sites, but also in the equine sited to ensure the mechanical efficiency of tendons, e.g. check ligaments.

To massage effectively it is essential to locate and avoid areas where bone protuberances lie just beneath the surface. They do, however, make useful skeletal landmarks as they provide pointers which aid in the location of muscle masses.

STRUCTURE OF HORSE'S SKIN

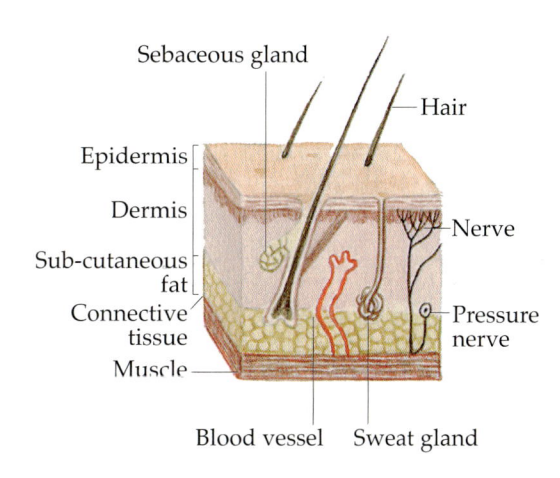

AREAS TO LOCATE THEN AVOID:

a Immediately behind ear; wing of atlas
b Just above throat; cervical (neck) vertebrae
c Spine of scapula
d Point of elbow; olecranon process
e Centrally behind knee; accessory carpal bone
f Ribs
g Centre of back; spinous processes of thoracic (back) vertebrae
h Stifle joint; patella
i Point of hip; tuber coxae
j Jumper's bump; tuber sacrale, highest point of pelvis

Circulatory and Lymphatic Systems

The body is described anatomically as consisting of 'systems', e.g. nervous, digestive. Each has a specific function but all must integrate; no 'one' can function independently.

The two systems considered to be responsive to massage are the venous section of the cardiovascular system, and the lymphatic system.

Circulatory System

This system circulates blood throughout the body via a complex network of vessels. It acts as a perpetual-motion conveyor belt driven by a pump, the heart; if the heart stops, the animal dies.

Arteries deliver nutrients and oxygen-rich blood to the body. Veins are the collectors, returning waste-laden blood to the appropriate sites.

Arterial walls are thick, built to withstand the pressure created by the pumping heart. Venous walls are thin and much more pliable; they are under considerably less pressure.

Veins rely on muscle activity to assist the return flow of the blood-borne waste to collecting points for either recycling or excretion.

Veins wend tortuous paths through tissue relying on internal valves to prevent blood back-flow.

Superficial veins are visible on the surface of a thin-skinned animal which is hot after exercise – make a point of observing this and try to visualise their all-embracing complexity. Press your finger along a vein, working toward the body centre and you can see the effect of the pressure you apply: the vein will swell in front of your finger and flatten behind; the vessel will then fill again as the finger pressure is removed.

Lymphatic System

This is a drainage system involved in the collection of waste, particularly that caused by injury or illness. Throughout the system are lymph nodes, clumps of specialist tissue called glands, designed to manufacture some of the cells required to combat infection.

Lymphatic vessels lie adjacent to many of the main veins, so pressure over the veins also affects lymph flow as it too moves slowly through its own network, working toward the body centre to empty into the thoracic duct.

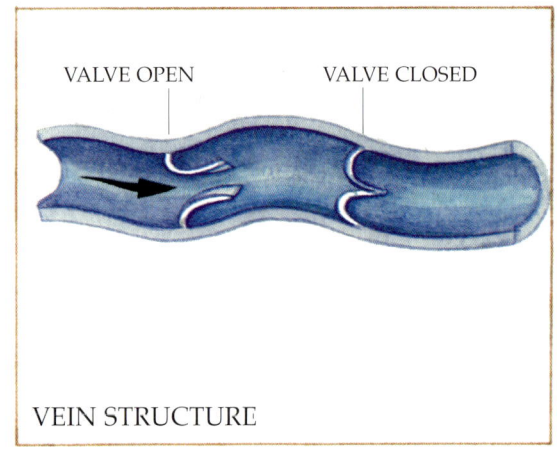

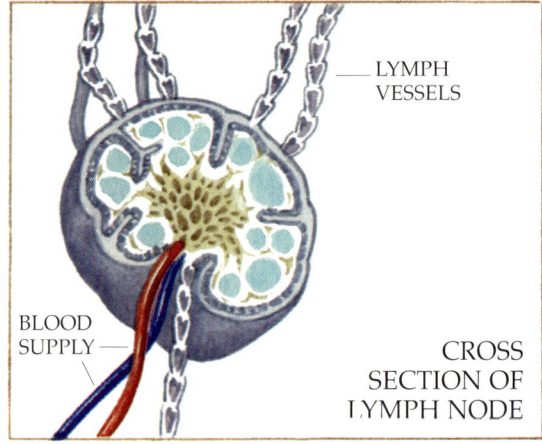

VALVE OPEN   VALVE CLOSED

VEIN STRUCTURE

LYMPH VESSELS

BLOOD SUPPLY

CROSS SECTION OF LYMPH NODE

CIRCULATORY SYSTEM

LYMPHATIC SYSTEM

All lymph vessels follow the pattern of the main veins, eventually discharging into a venous vessel – the thoracic duct.

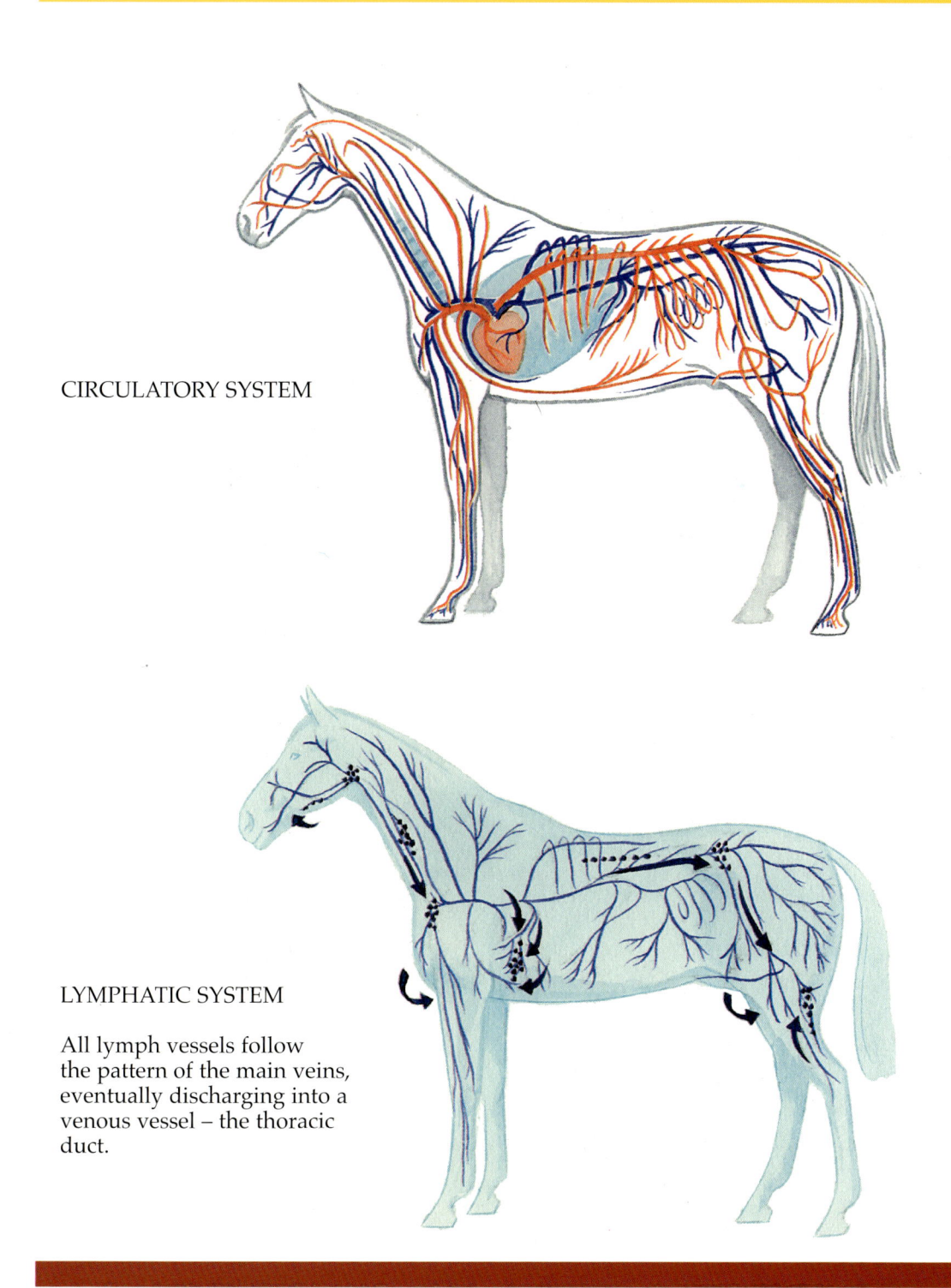

Massage Techniques

Effleurage (stroking)
The technique can be double- or single-handed. The stroke direction should follow the course of the major veins. Start distally (away) from the central body mass, work proximally (inward) toward the central body mass.

The hands should *mould* to the underlying contours. The operator's body weight is used to exert pressure as the hands are first pushed away, then drawn gently back without pressure to position for the next stroke.

Work lightly at first, increasing pressure as the animal relaxes.

Effects:
- Enhances venous and lymphatic flow.
- Promotes relaxation.

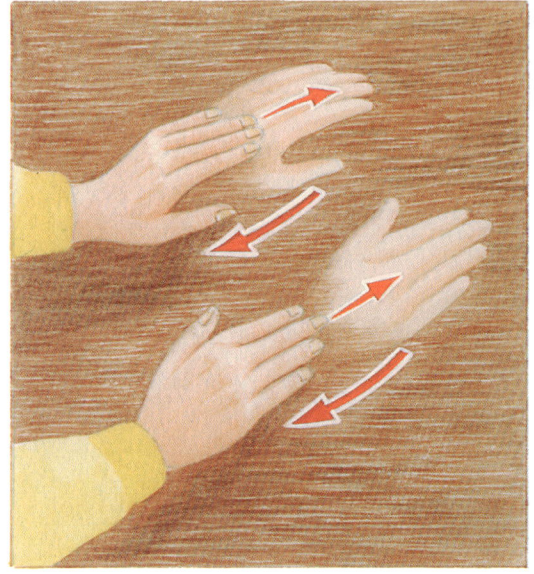

Palms and fingers mould to the underlying surface. Push away exerting pressure, draw lightly back, or vice versa.

Petrissage (compression)
This is a double-handed technique. The underlying soft tissues are grasped lightly between fingers, heel of the hands and thumbs, picked up (hands working alternately) squeezed gently and returned to their resting position.

Effects:
- Mobilises tissue.
- Improves circulatory flow with alternating compression and relaxation.
- Influences deep-tissue vessels.

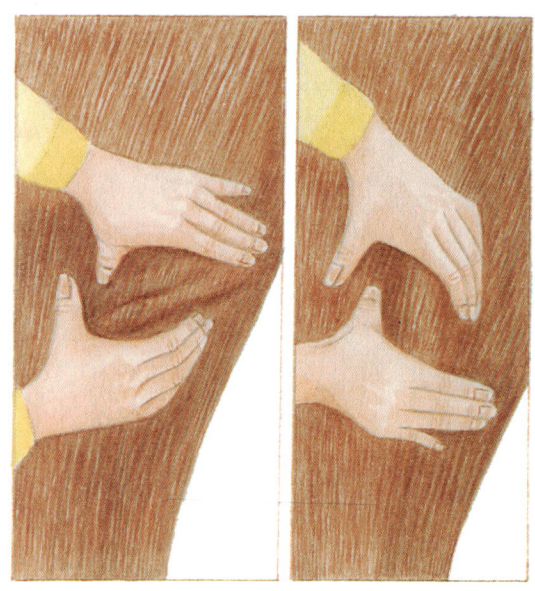

Hands alternately gather sections of muscle, grip lightly, squeeze, release and repeat.

Tapotment (percussion)

The following three techniques are usually double handed.

The operator's hands are clenched into loose fists. The little finger sides of the fists bounce alternately on and off the underlying muscle mass.

To achieve the required effect movement takes place in the wrists and forearms. Loose fists are held with the fingers toward each other, thumbs up. As one hand rotates down to meet the surface so the other rotates up.

Effects:
- Muscle contraction followed by relaxation, achieving enhanced circulatory flow.
- A vibratory effect leading to muscle relaxation.

Only suitable for large muscle masses.

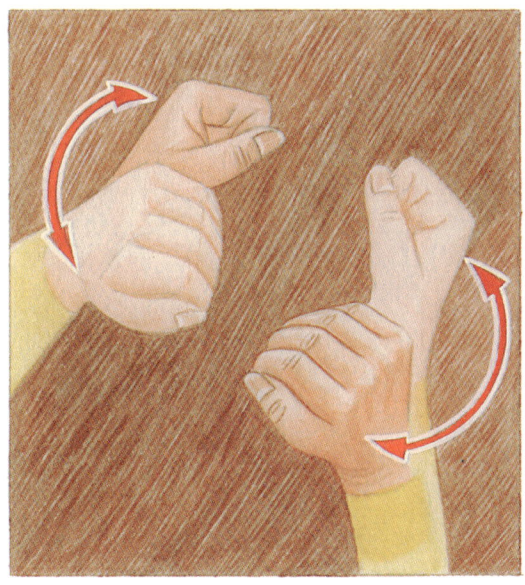

Loosely clenched fists bounce on the underlying tissue.

Kneading

This is a single- or double-handed technique.

To knead using the hand, the fingers are clenched into a fist, the backs of the fingers and knuckles press deep down into the muscle mass, twisting slightly at the end of the compression before releasing. The movement can be likened to kneading/beating dough.

A finger, reinforced by a second, can be used in a circular manner to affect small localised areas where the whole hand will not fit.

Effects:
- Compression and relaxation influences deep-sited vessels.

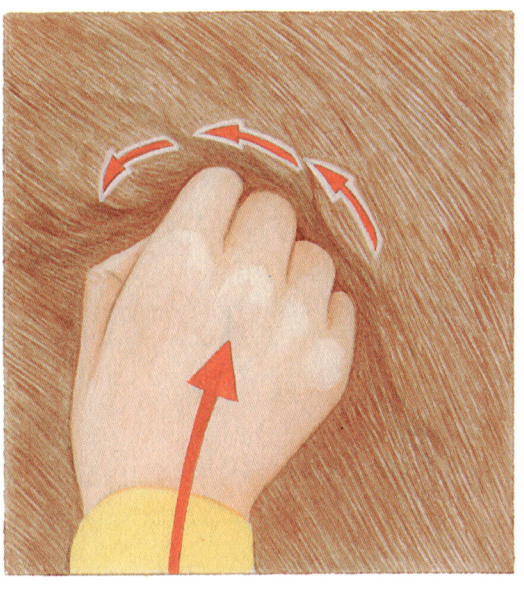

The backs of the fingers and knuckles press down into the muscle, twisting slightly before releasing.

Massage Techniques (cont.)

Clapping
The hands are cupped, the tips of the fingers maintain loose contact with the surface. The cupped hands lift and drop alternately as the operator's wrists flex and extend.

Effects:
- Stimulation of surface vessels.
- Applied briskly, can be used to stimulate the whole body following relaxation.

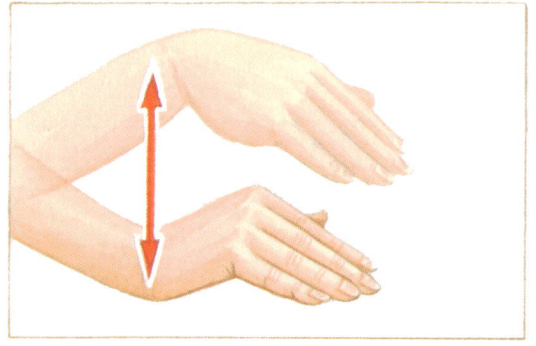

A loosely cupped hand is made by lifting and dropping the wrist. The sound should resemble the 'plop' of a stone in water.

Hacking
The hands are turned sideways to the underlying surface, palms facing each other.
  By rotating the forearms alternately, the little finger sides of the hands drop onto the surface and bounce off.

Effects:
- As clapping. Useful in confined areas or over small muscle masses.

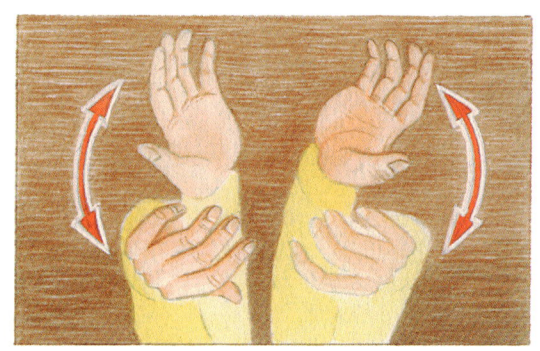

A stimulation technique achieved by rotation of the wrists allowing the sides and backs of fingers to meet the surface.

Friction
This is a single-handed technique.
  The tip of one finger, reinforced by the second, is placed firmly over the area targeted. With the **skin moving as one** with the working fingertip, the masseur works **across, not with,** the underlying fibre direction.

Effect:
- To create a greatly increased circulation in a very local area.

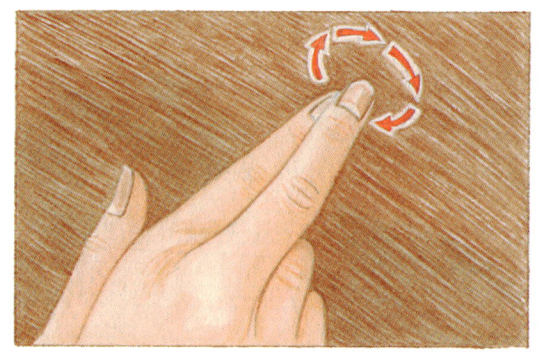

The underlying finger, reinforced by the second, works across the underlying fibres. The skin must move as one with the finger.

Massage Equipment

Soft plastic pads, bath mitts, cactus cloth gloves, and reversible rubber gloves with a stiff bristle pad on one side and rubber bushes on the opposite, are available in tack stores classed as massage aids.

Their main disadvantages are that the masseur cannot 'feel' what is happening under the hands, and that the intimate communication between operator's hands and horse's body is lost.

The most useful are probably the 'bath mitts'. Used gently behind the elbow, inside the stifle and under the jaw, they are often tolerated better than the hand and achieve relaxation, allowing for a better result of the total body massage.

Mechanical Massagers

These can be both hand held or specially designed as pads which 'sit' over the horse's back; they vibrate.
Pain research demonstrates that continuous vibration delivered at a specific frequency will, after varying periods of time, reduce pain sensation.

The length of time required for this effect varies and is dependent both upon the frequency of vibration and cause of pain.

There is little evidence to demonstrate any other effects.

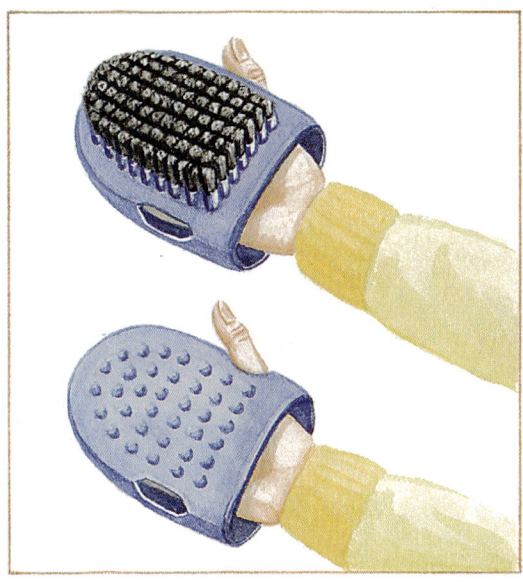

Gloves and aids are available but intimate contact is lost with their use.

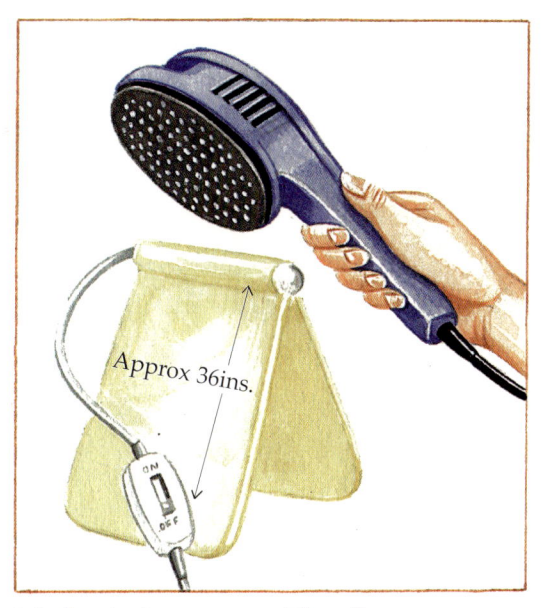

Mechanical massagers. The effects are vibratory and as such can help to reduce local discomfort.

Body Massage

Effleurage sites and stroke direction for all techniques.

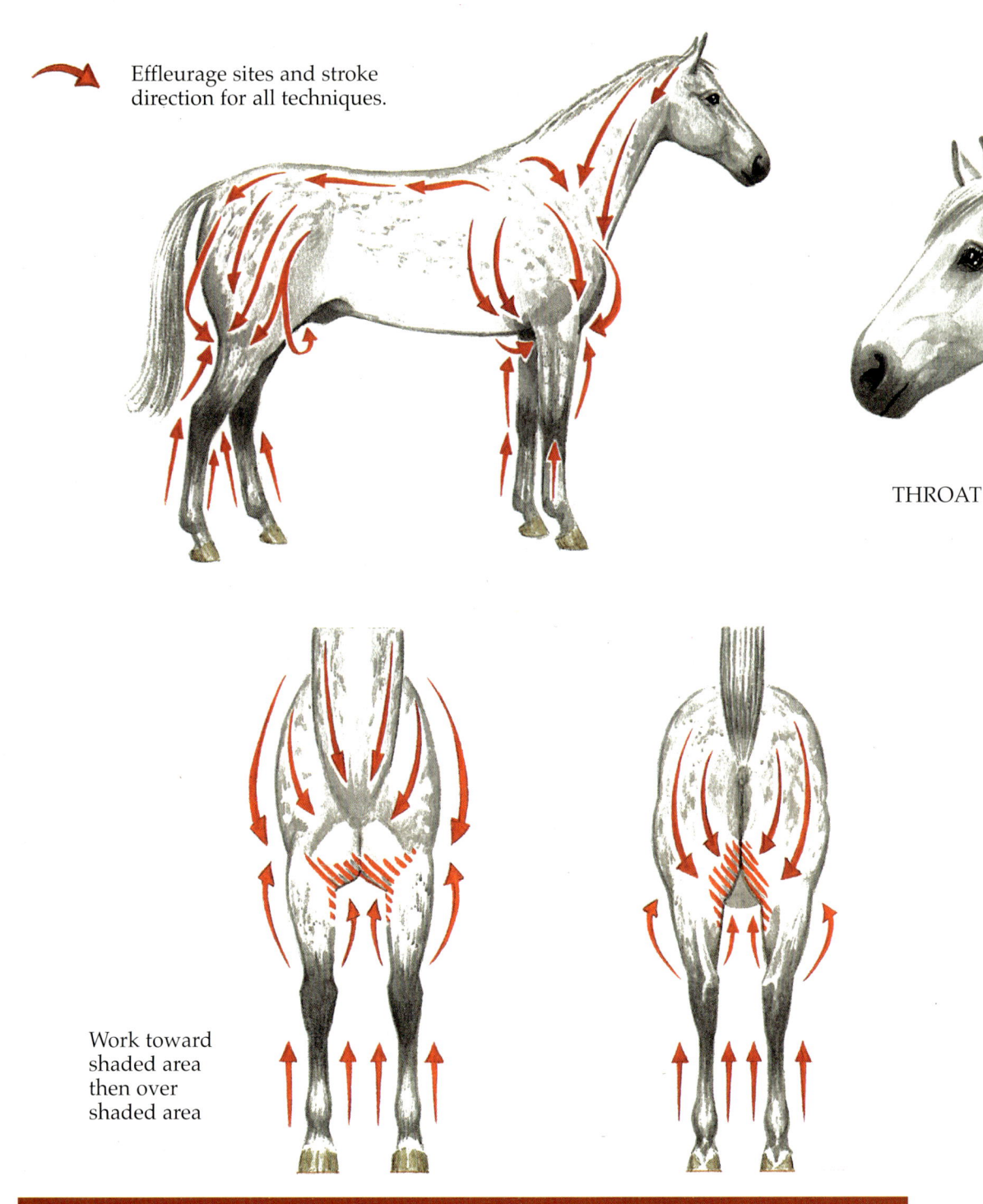

THROAT

Work toward shaded area then over shaded area

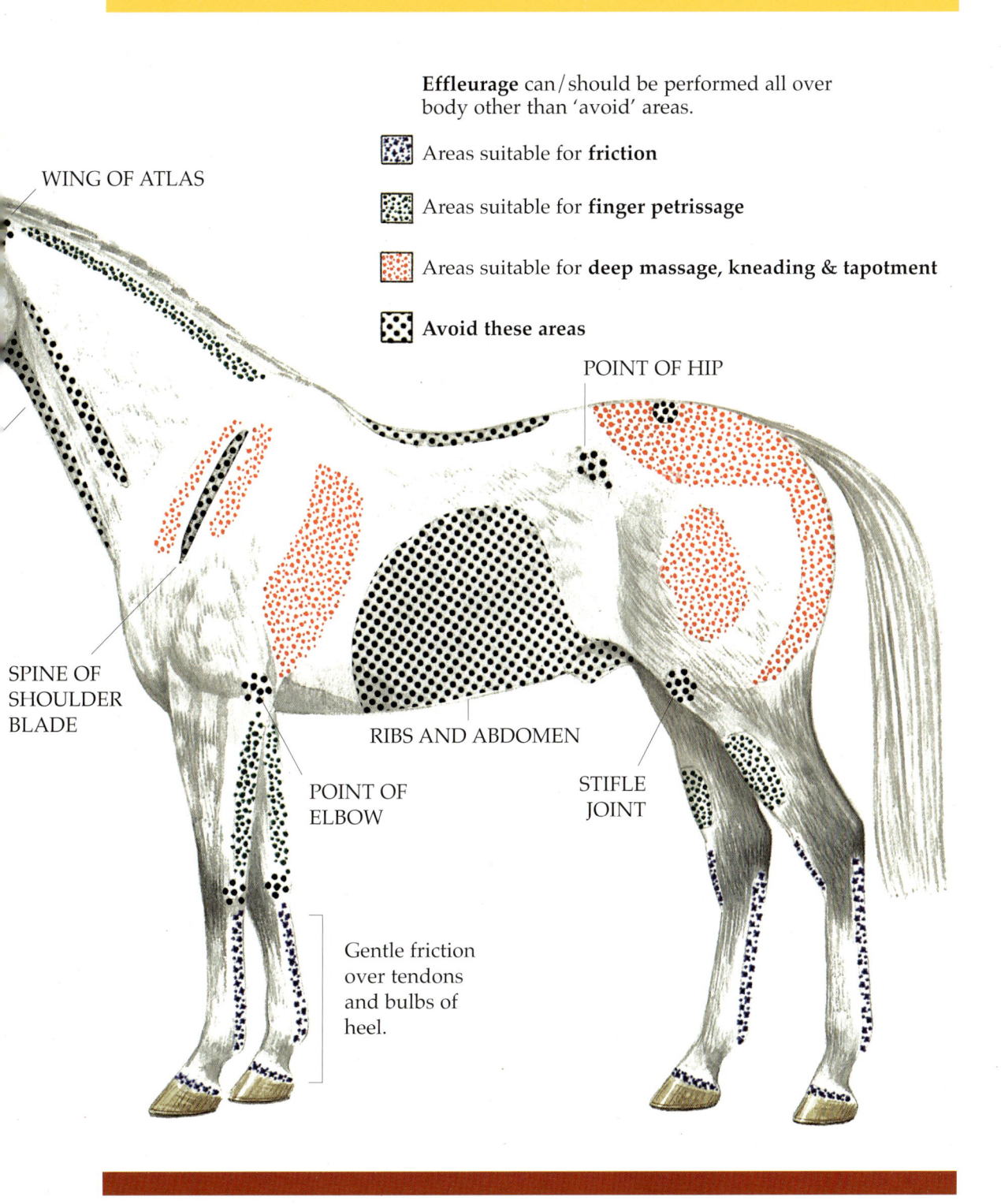

Effleurage can/should be performed all over body other than 'avoid' areas.

- Areas suitable for **friction**
- Areas suitable for **finger petrissage**
- Areas suitable for **deep massage, kneading & tapotment**
- Avoid these areas

WING OF ATLAS

POINT OF HIP

SPINE OF SHOULDER BLADE

RIBS AND ABDOMEN

POINT OF ELBOW

STIFLE JOINT

Gentle friction over tendons and bulbs of heel.

13

Body Massage (cont.)

Routine

Tie the horse loosely and make certain that the stall is free of hazards, i.e. floor feed bowls, half buried mineral blocks.

Let the horse smell your hands, then stroke the neck gently and let the horse smell your hands again – it will begin to relax at its own familiar scent.

Run your hands lightly all over the animal's body as the arrows direct.

If the horse is tall stand on a box or milk crate to achieve height.

Begin your massage with light effleurage, starting from behind the ears and slowly working the body section by section, as follows:

• Nearside: neck, shoulder area, chest, back, hindquarters, near fore, near hind.

• Offside: neck, shoulder area, chest, back, hindquarters, off fore, off hind.

Increase the effleurage pressure as the animal relaxes. Incorporate other techniques over muscle masses, section by section.

Finish with effleurage, again working section by section.

If **relaxation** is the aim, do *not* use hacking or clapping.

If **stimulation** is required, at the conclusion of the final effleurage hack/clap the entire torso.

All horses should have a full body massage pre-competition.

The main areas of stress for each discipline require particular attention and this can be given during a post-competition massage. (See individual sports on following pages.)

A full body massage takes approximately 45 minutes.

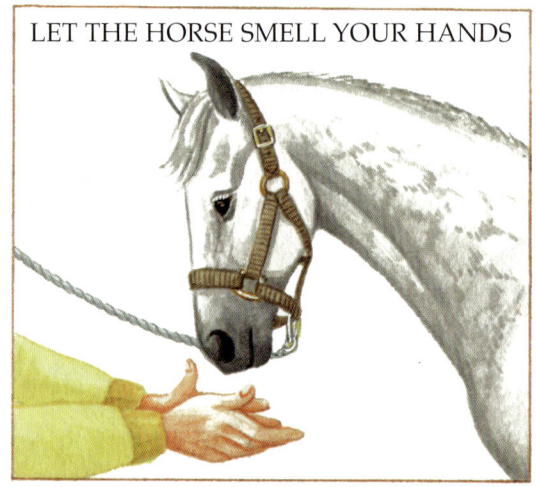

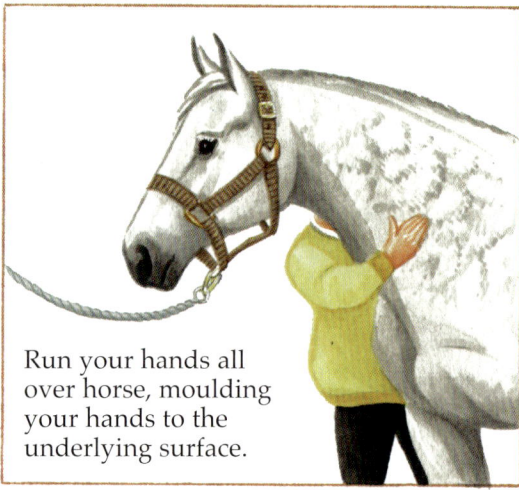

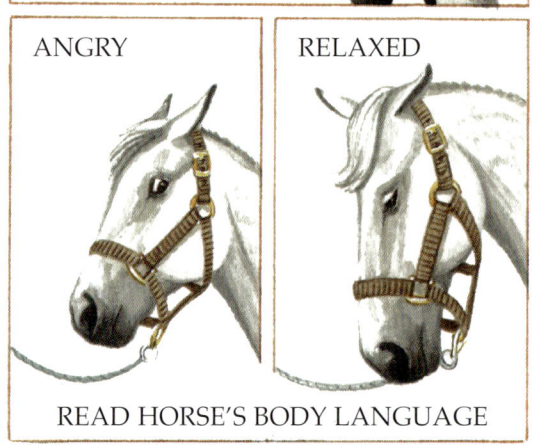

LET THE HORSE SMELL YOUR HANDS

Run your hands all over horse, moulding your hands to the underlying surface.

ANGRY

RELAXED

READ HORSE'S BODY LANGUAGE

Use your body weight.

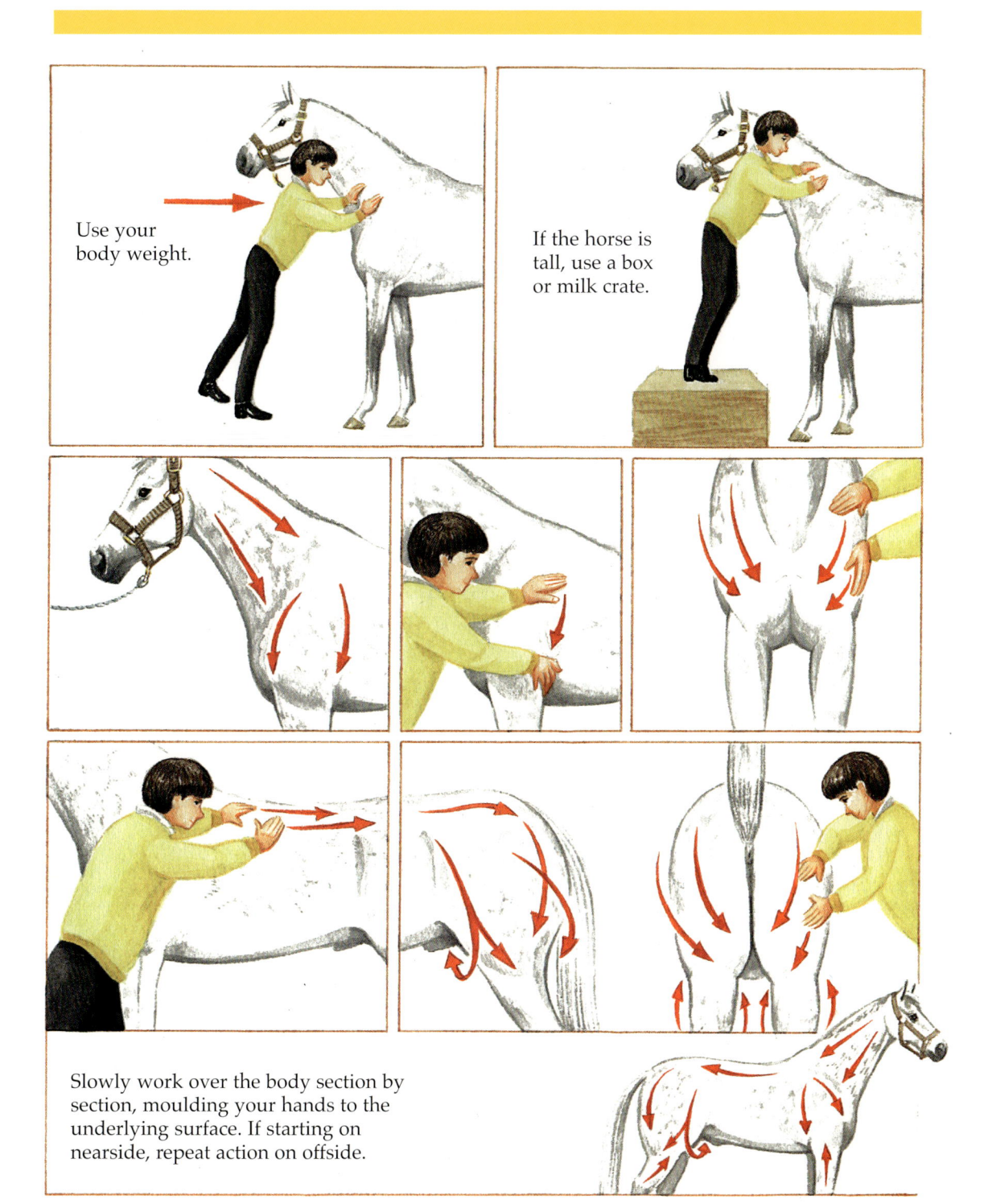

If the horse is tall, use a box or milk crate.

Slowly work over the body section by section, moulding your hands to the underlying surface. If starting on nearside, repeat action on offside.

15

The Pleasure Horse

Pleasure and general riding requirements vary, dependent upon location and demands.

An important point to remember is that in many cases the exercise undertaken by these horses tends to follow an irregular pattern, sometimes with excessive weekend work, rather than a regular level of activity.

The equine back is a multi-jointed rod held together by ligaments. It is supported in a rather inadequate manner by muscles located not only along the back but also over the quarters and in front of the rib cage.

Back ache, resulting from activity, is common in partially fit humans and horses. Man can rub the aching area; the horse must resort to rolling. In a confined space this can result in the animal getting cast, often acquiring an unnecessary injury.

To avoid this, all casually ridden horses should have their backs massaged before and after exercise.

Refer to appropriate disciplines if the animal is schooled or jumped.

Stress areas

- Back, from mid neck to mid quarters
  ⇨ Effleurage, petrissage, hacking/clapping

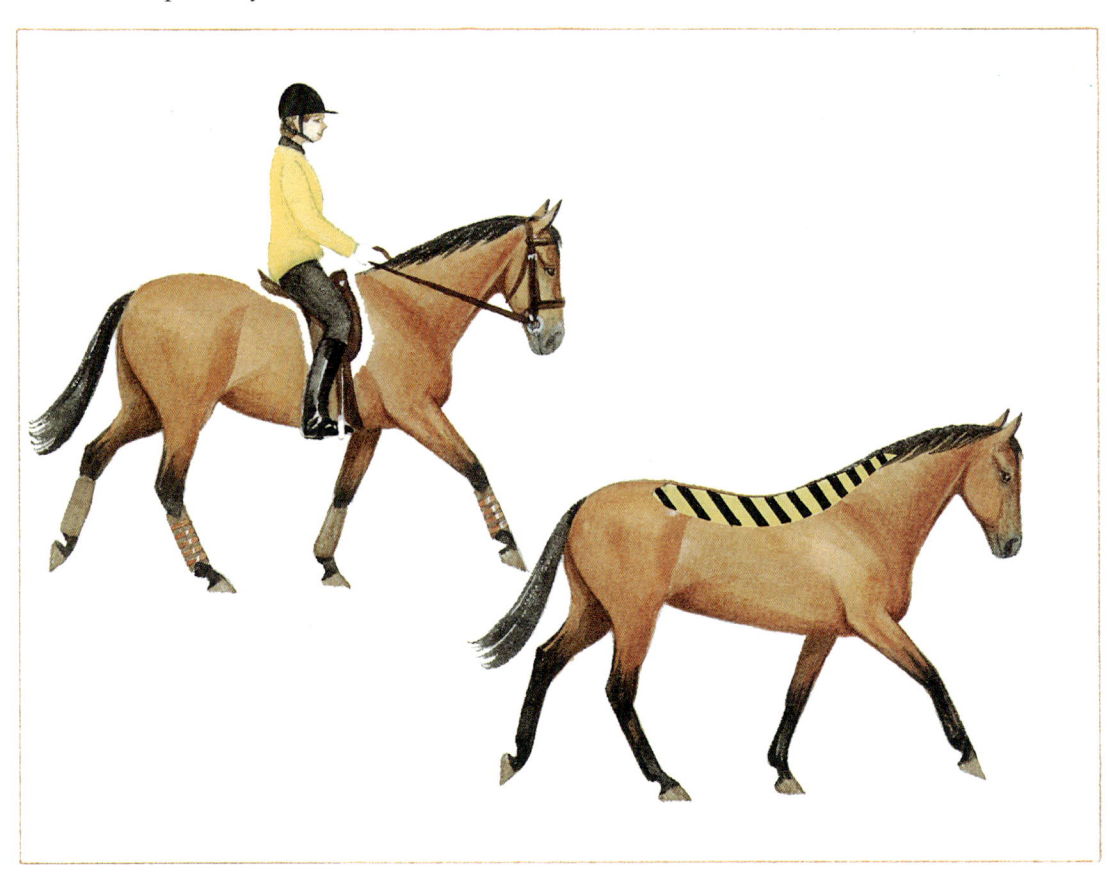

Dressage

The dressage horse is trained to perform a series of complicated changes of gait including lateral work. The head and neck must not move and total balance is essential. Much of the work necessitates muscle activity in the most tiring range. The static positioning of head and neck involves crucifying tension in that area. In advanced tests the stress levels to hock and stifle are incalculable.

The discipline is probably the most exhausting for muscles, also the most mentally and physically demanding of all equine disciplines.

Competition stress areas

- Poll ⇨ Finger petrissage
- Behind the jaw ⇨ Finger petrissage
- Withers ⇨ Finger petrissage
- Loins ⇨ Gentle hacking
- Forearm ⇨ Effleurage
- Inner side of front legs onto chest ⇨ Effleurage
- Hamstrings ⇨ Effleurage
- Second thigh ⇨ Finger petrissage
- Inner sides of hind legs ⇨ Effleurage

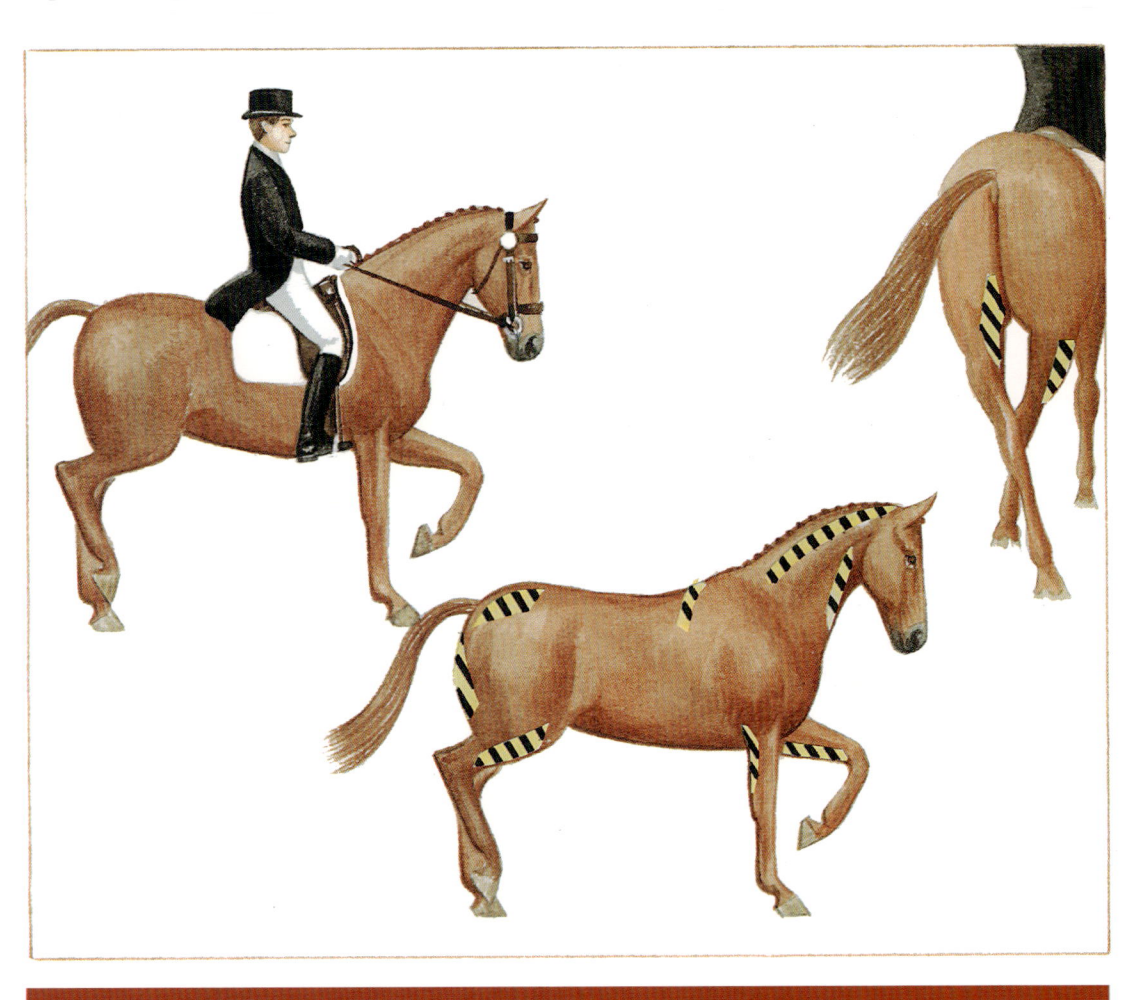

Endurance Riding

Endurance horses must be able to negotiate long distances over varying terrain. The sport has developed in a manner which necessitates riding at moderate speeds over calculated distances, not enabling the horse to utilise ligamentous loading, a feature which is designed to assist the muscles and reduce fatigue, and associated only with fast extended paces.

The sport requires a fit rider *not* a passenger.

Competition stress areas

- Back, from withers to loins
  ⇨ Effleurage/clapping
- Muscles of the shoulders
  ⇨ Effleurage, petrissage
- Muscles of the forearm ⇨ Effleurage
- Muscles of the second thigh
  ⇨ Effleurage

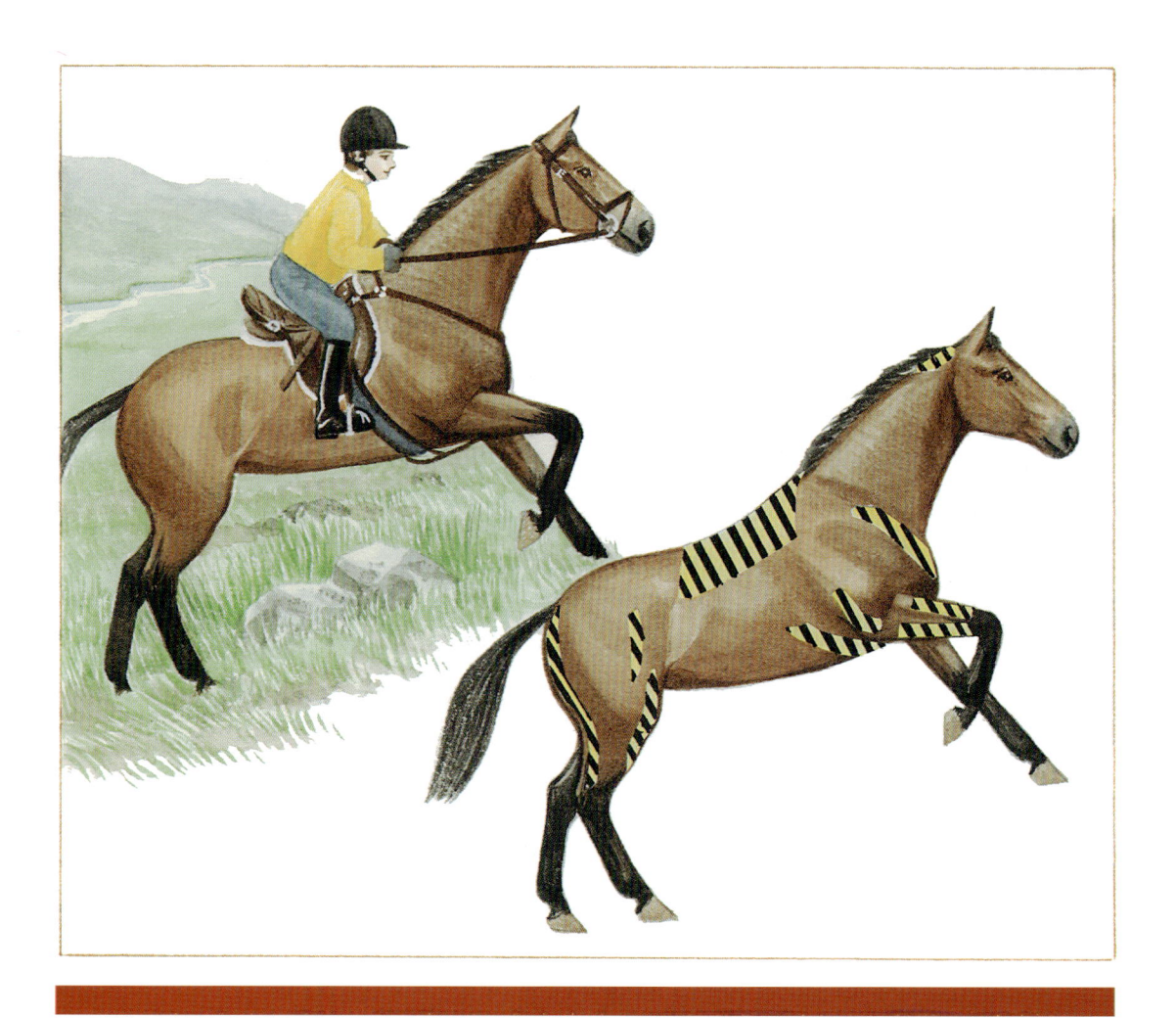

Driving

The unnatural position of the horse's head and neck, the need to balance a wheeled vehicle, to lean into the collar or breast plate to pull, then lean back into the breeching to brake, demands a very complex muscular co-ordination with tremendous strain transmitted to the mid-back.

As most of the work is 'collected', muscle activity is in the mid or most tiring range.

Competition stress areas

- Just behind the poll ⇨ Finger petrissage
- Shoulders
  ⇨ Effleurage, finger petrissage
- Forearm ⇨ Effleurage
- Mid-back ⇨ Finger petrissage, hacking
- Quarters ⇨ Effleurage, kneading
- Second thigh
  ⇨ Effleurage and petrissage

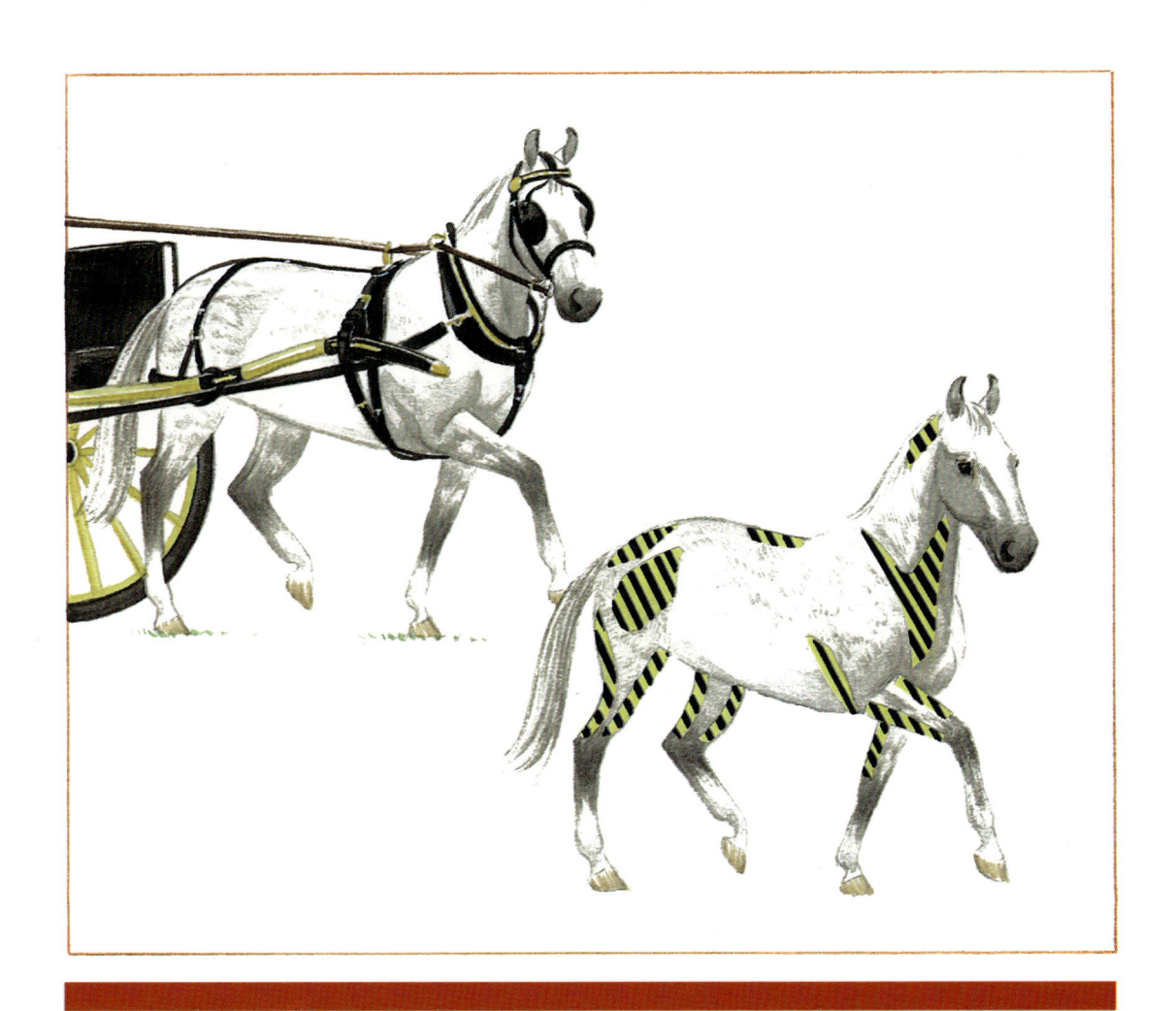

Show Jumping

Show jumping demands sudden explosive spurts of energy, mostly in the middle range of muscle activity.

Full extension is only required if a water jump is included. Against the clock, it is the inside hindleg that suffers in every turn.

As the horse leaves the ground it is the hindquarters that achieve propulsion, and although the leading front leg is the first to reach the ground it remains there as a *prop* only, for it is the leading hindleg that takes the strain of the full body weight as the animal lands. In show jumping each round must be assessed so that if the course favours one direction, you can concentrate on the leg affected.

Competition stress areas

- Hind legs
  ⇨ Effleurage, petrissage
- Loins
  ⇨ Effleurage, hacking/cupping

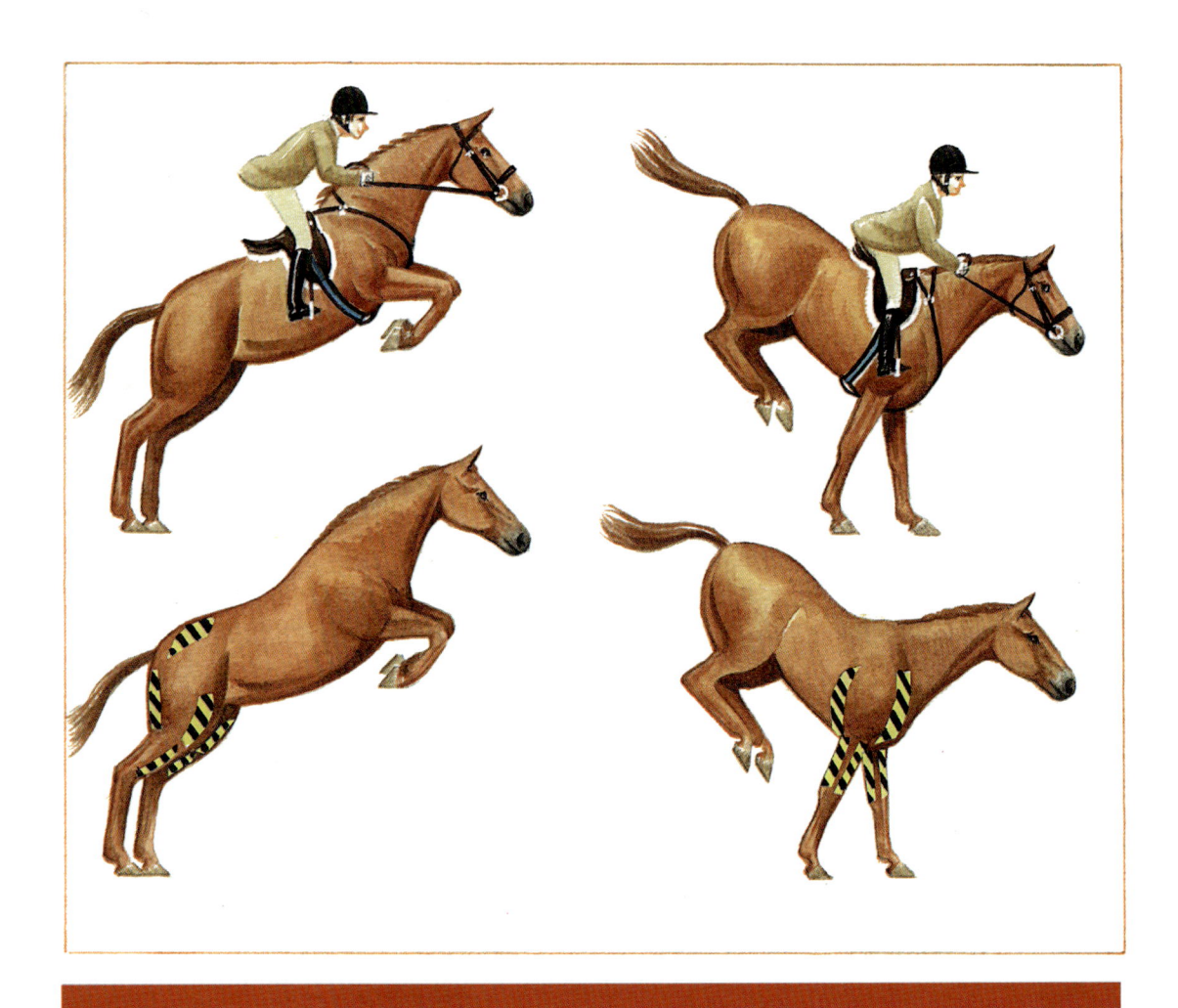

Cross-Country

Cross-country events include team chasing, hunter trials, and eventing. The latter involves competing in three disciplines, either all in one day or spread over a two- or three-day period. Jumping and galloping are a feature of all. In fast work such as this, muscle activity is aided by the fact that the animal can supplement muscular effort with ligamentous loading.

Provided the competing animal has been prepared for the task, a general body massage before and after the competition is the most beneficial approach.

Should a fall or other accident occur the muscle groups stressed during the mishap deserve special attention. For example, if a horse lands badly, falls and bends its neck sideways, massage the muscles on the side that hit the ground first and were stretched as the neck was bent in an unnatural manner.

So, read the fall and address the appropriate areas.

Competition stress areas

- Dependent upon types of jump, number of hills, ground conditions and falls
  ⇨ Use a general body approach

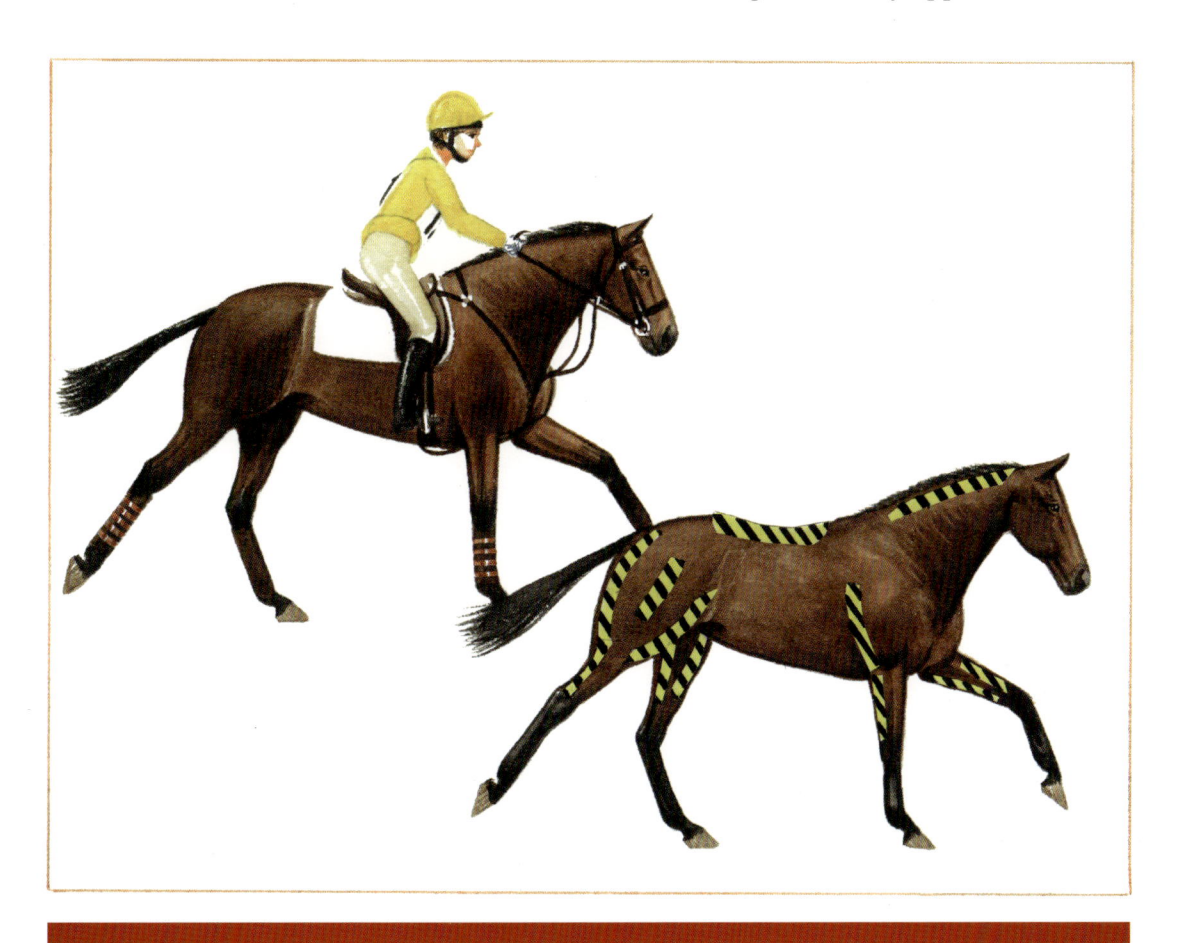

Ice Massage

Competition, no matter what the discipline, often results in minor tissue damage, not severe enough to warrant veterinary intervention but requiring care and attention. Ice is the most useful tool in situations where the horse has had a knock down while jumping, hit a pole hard, bruised a shin or joint, has been kicked, has a muscle bruise, a boot rub or other localised soft tissue trauma.

Effects of ice

1 Constriction of local vessels allowing any damaged area to 'seal off'.

2 Reduction in local metabolic (cellular) activity, reducing the need for local oxygen.

3 An increase, after approximately 20 minutes, of circulatory flow within deep vessels in the area, as the thermo-regulators signal the area is too cold. ('Hunters' Rush')

Application

• For small areas, massage with an ice cube on a 'lolly' stick for 15-20 minutes. Leave 2-3 hour gaps between applications.

• For larger areas, massage with ice cubes in a plastic bag. Rub gently over the area for 15-20 minutes every 2-3 hours.

NB: Over-chilling an area negates all the required effects.

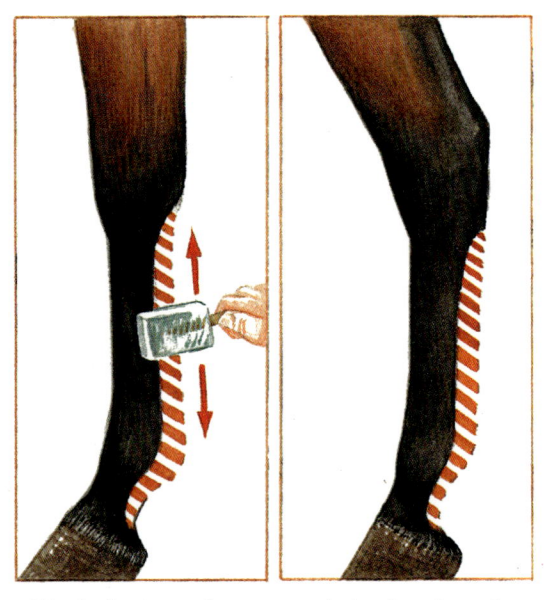

Work the ice cube upwards both sides of the leg. Bandage in between applications.

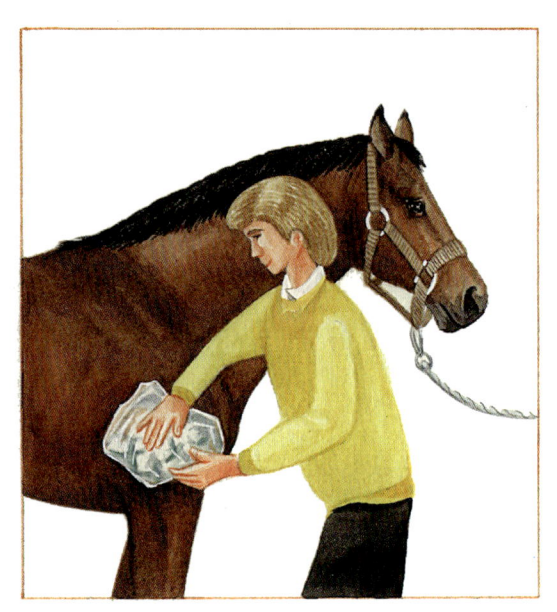

Rub gently around the area of swelling in a circular motion.

Teaching and Strengthening the Hands

Most people are predominantly right or left handed. A lucky few are ambidextrous. To massage well both hands must work together.

Tension
To appreciate the difference between tension and relaxation hold an apple in one hand (firm, crisp variety) and an orange in the other. With the eyes closed squeeze both: a tense muscle feels like the apple; a relaxed muscle feels like the orange. Change the fruits from hand to hand. Concentrate on the difference in tension.

Strength and Flexibility
Sensitive, strong yet flexible hands are essential for the masseur. The following hand exercises can help to develop these qualities. Exercise both hands at the same time.

1 Stretch the fingers as though trying to span an octave. Close to a loose fist. Repeat several times.

2 With the palms face up, circle both thumbs clockwise and anticlockwise.

3 Shake both hands for relaxation.

4 Using a rubber band, open and close the fingers against the resistance of the band. The higher up the fingers, the greater the resistance.

5 To exercise the thumb, move the thumb away from the finger against the resistance of the band.

6 Squeeze a squash or tennis ball, holding one of a similar resistance in each hand.

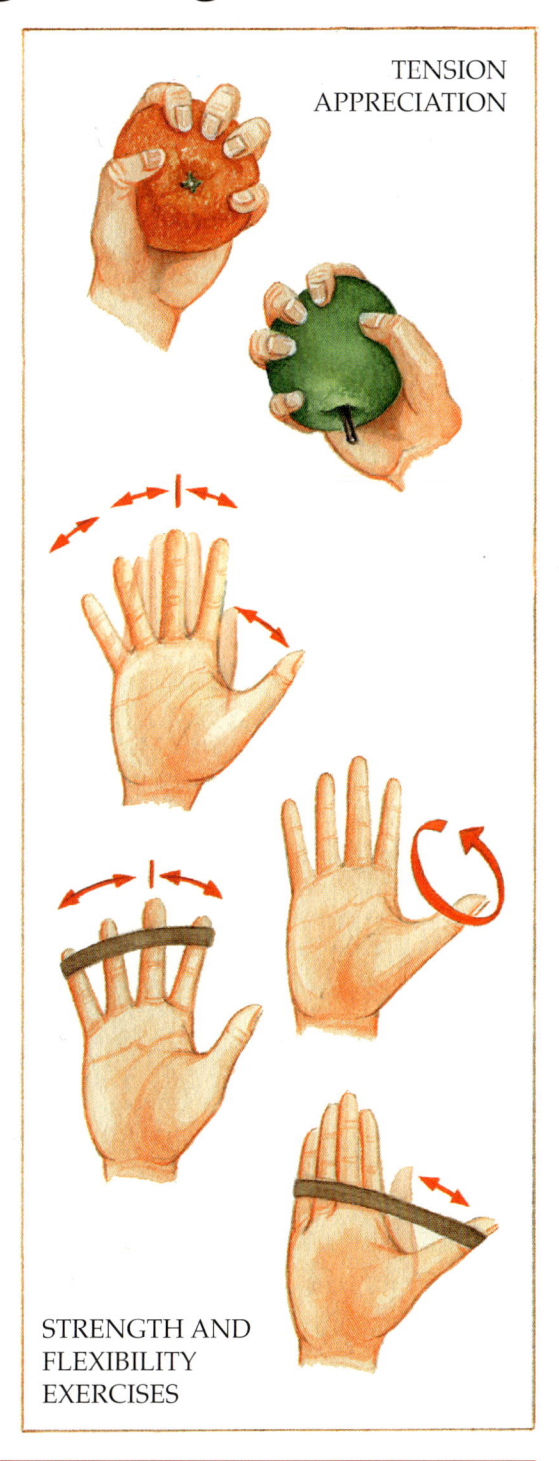

TENSION APPRECIATION

STRENGTH AND FLEXIBILITY EXERCISES

Indications for Massage

The massage techniques described in the previous pages are designed to prepare the horse for competition, via a *full body massage*, then to assist recovery after competition (see the *stress areas* for differing disciplines).

Contra-indications
Do not apply massage to:
- a horse that has tied up.
- a very lame horse that has not been seen by a veterinary surgeon.
- a horse suffering any infection, local or general.
- a horse with lymphangitis.
- a horse with any skin condition/eruption, e.g. ringworm.
- a horse with any undiagnosed abnormality.

This book does not set out to discuss therapeutic (medical) massage, acupressure, shiatsu, connective tissue massage. While all employ massage techniques each is a specialist subject requiring in-depth study.

It is a legal offence for any person to practise massage on an animal owned by another person without the permission of a veterinary surgeon, normally the veterinary surgeon who would attend the animal in question. (Veterinary Surgeons Act, 1966)

It is assumed that persons practising the described massage techniques are fully aware of the risks associated with work around horses.

The author and publisher are not responsible for any injury sustained by persons attempting to massage, neither can they be held responsible for any injury resulting from the inappropriate use of massage.

Persons interested in furthering their knowledge can obtain details of books and courses from: The Secretary, Downs House, Baydon, SN8 2JS, England.